WEIGHT LOSS

FORMAT FOR

2024

HOW TO CREATE A HEALTHY LIFESTYLE

THAT ALLOWS YOU TO SYSTEMATICALLY

LOSE WEIGHT IN THE MOST ACCURATE AND

POSSIBLE WAY

BY

LAUREL M. BOWMAN

TABLE OF CONTENTS

INTRODUCTION

Within the realms of medicine, health, and physical fitness, weight loss signifies a decrease in overall body mass resulting from a reduction in fluid retention, body fat (adipose tissue), or lean mass, which includes bone mineral density, muscle, tendon, and related connective tissues is referred to as weight loss in the contexts of health, fitness, and medicine.

Weight loss can occur unintentionally as a result of malnourishment or an underlying condition, or it can occur as a result of a conscious endeavor to better an actual or perceived overweight or obese state. Cachexia is defined as "unexplained" weight loss that is not induced by a reduction in caloric intake or an increase in exercise and may be a symptom of a serious medical condition.

The loss of total body mass as a result of efforts to enhance fitness and health or to change appearance through shrinking is referred to as intentional weight loss. Weight loss is the primary treatment for obesity, and there is significant evidence that a 7-10% weight loss will prevent progression from prediabetes to type 2 diabetes and manage cardiometabolic health in diabetics with a 5-15% weight loss.

Weight loss among individuals dealing with overweight or obesity can significantly mitigate health risks, enhance fitness levels, and delay the onset of diabetes. Moreover, it holds promise in alleviating discomfort and fostering mobility for individuals afflicted by knee osteoarthritis. While weight loss can effectively lower hypertension (high blood pressure), its impact on reducing hypertension-related damage remains uncertain. Achieving weight loss involves adopting a lifestyle that prioritizes consuming fewer calories than expended. Factors such as depression, stress, or boredom can contribute to weight gain, necessitating medical attention for those experiencing these circumstances.

According to a 2010 study, dieters who got a full night's sleep shed more than twice as much weight as those who didn't. Though vitamin D supplementation may be beneficial, This is not supported by research. Long-term trends indicate that most individuals who engage in dieting eventually regain weight. Those who acquire and maintain a healthy weight, according to the UK National Health Service and the Dietary Guidelines for Americans, do so most successfully by consuming only enough calories to meet their needs and being physically active. Changes in food and lifestyle must be permanent for weight loss to be permanent. There is evidence that counseling or exercise alone do not result in weight loss, whereas dieting alone leads in significant long-term weight loss, and a combination of dieting and exercise results in the best results. Meal replacements, orlistat, a very low-calorie diet, and extensive primary care physician intervention can all help with considerable weight loss.

1

CAUSES OF OBESITY AND OVERWEIGHT

What factors contribute to obesity and overweight?

Multiple factors play a role in both acquiring and sustaining excess weight. Diet, sedentary lifestyle, environmental factors, and genetic predisposition are all illustrative instances. Some of these factors are briefly explored in the next section. More information on the causes of overweight and obesity can be found at the National Heart, Lung, and Blood Institute.

Food addiction and Activity

Numerous sugar-laden and high-fat processed foods activate the reward centers in your brain.. These foods are frequently compared to commonly misused drugs such as alcohol, cocaine, nicotine, and cannabis. Junk foods can lead to addiction in vulnerable people. These people lose control over their eating habits, just as persons suffering from alcoholism lose control over their drinking habits.

Addiction is a complicated problem that can be very challenging to resolve. When you develop an addiction, your brain's biochemistry takes over and you lose your ability to make decisions for yourself.

The availability of food has expanded substantially over the past few centuries, which is another element that has a significant impact on people's waistlines. stuff is omnipresent these days, especially junk stuff. Stores put appetizing foods where you are most likely to notice them.

Another issue is that, particularly in America, junk food is sometimes less expensive than complete, healthful diets. Some people don't even have the choice of buying actual goods, such fresh fruit and vegetables, especially in impoverished areas. In some locations, the only items sold at convenience stores are sodas, candies, and packaged, processed junk food. Weight gain occurs as a result of consuming more calories than the body expends through physical activity—an imbalance that stands as the primary driver of increased weight

Environment

Our ability to maintain a healthy weight is influenced by the environment in which we live. For instance: It is difficult for people to be physically active when there aren't any nearby parks, sidewalks, or reasonably priced gyms.

• Americans consume more calories from oversized meal portions, which means they need to engage in even more physical activity to maintain a healthy weight.

• Food advertising pushes consumers to purchase unhealthy meals like sugary drinks and high-fat snacks;

• Some people lack access to shops that offer reasonably priced, healthful foods like fresh fruits and vegetables.1.

Genetics

Studies indicate that genetics contributes to obesity. Obesity can be directly caused by genes in conditions like Prader-Willi syndrome.

Genetics may also play a role in an individual's propensity to gain weight. Researchers think that while a person's genetics may make them more likely to be obese, other factors—like having an abundance of food or not getting enough exercise—may also be necessary for someone to be overweight.

Health Conditions and Medications

Overweight and obesity can be brought on by certain hormone issues, such as polycystic ovarian syndrome, Cushing syndrome, and underactive thyroid.

A number of medications, such as certain corticosteroids, antidepressants, and seizure medications, might also make you gain weight.

Stress, Emotional Factors, and Poor Sleep

Feelings of boredom, anger, distress, or stress can lead certain individuals to engage in overeating.

Additionally, research has shown that individuals are more likely to be overweight or obese the less sleep they get. This is partially due to the fact that hormones generated while you sleep regulate hunger and energy expenditure.

2

CHANGE YOUR MIND AND LOSE WEIGHT

It may seem unbelievable, but your body is not where effective weight loss starts. It goes beyond just cutting back on food and increasing exercise. It goes beyond simply counting calories in and out. Effective weight loss starts with a mental rather than a physical approach; it is more about how much you support and love yourself than it is about how hard you labor and starve your body. Therefore, in order for weight loss to be successful, it must start within—that is, in your heart, mind, and spirit. You won't be able to shed those excess pounds until you begin to love yourself without conditions and treat yourself with kindness, compassion, and care.

and prevent them from going. With the help of forty-two straightforward but effective techniques—such as mindful eating exercises, mind-body visualizations, and guided meditations—Mind-Body Weight Loss walks you through the inner journey to permanently losing weight. You will discover how to establish a positive, new relationship with food and with yourself as you put these ideas into practice. You'll discover how to release yourself from the grip of self-criticism, embrace and communicate your suppressed emotions, relieve tension, value your physical appearance, rekindle old connections, and find closure on long-standing family matters. Most significantly, though, you'll discover how to adopt a fresh viewpoint on your life and your circumstances

difficulties losing weight. With a broader and more intelligent viewpoint, you will be able to see your overindulgence in food differently and identify the strategies that work best for you to lose weight and keep it off. Most people start with food and exercise (or supplements or other goods meant for internal use) while attempting to reduce weight.

While eating well and exercising are unquestionably significant parts of any successful weight loss plan, it's also critical to remember that the mind is an important instrument.

Simply said, mindfulness can help you lose weight and improve your general health by managing your stress, attitude, and perspective. It can also help you avoid gaining weight or even lose a considerable amount of weight.

You can regulate your response to everyday life's events, including the stressful ones, by practicing mindfulness. Too much time is wasted by many fretting about the past or the uncertain future.

This is a normal reaction to the subconscious ideas that we form as a result of our experiences in life, but it has a significant effect on stress, health, and even weight.

Stress has a significant impact on weight in ways other than "stress eating." Cortisol, a hormone meant to shield the body from perceived danger, is released by the body in response to stress. This is advantageous when there is a genuine threat.

The issue is that cortisol is also frequently released when t here is no physical threat, which might happen when we ar e really anxious about an excessively busy schedule, issues with family or work, or other causes.

Furthermore, cortisol is known to contribute to extra abdo minal fat, maybe as an attempt to shield the organs from i magined threats.

On the other hand, when we learn to limit our thoughts to the things that we can manage right now, we can keep our emotions in check and avoid needless stress and the dama ge it causes to our bodies.

Limiting your thoughts only teaches you more efficient me thods to deal with life's facts, not that you have to ignore them to handle significant problems. And with enough practice, this is quite doable because humans have the ability to alter the way they think.

Gaining awareness in all areas of life can be quite advantageous for your weight loss endeavors. We may enhance our general health and lifespan by using mind-body connection techniques like mindfulness, self-compassion, and meditation. We can also avoid or reduce weight gain. We believe that willpower is much overvalued! In any weight loss program, the first necessary step is mind training, not willpower. More than our physical health, we must teach our minds to be disciplined and persistently motivate ourselves.

Taking the initiative to create a healthy diet can tip the scales in your favor. Once you are in the appropriate mindset, you'll be astounded at how simple it is to adhere to the nutrition regimens!

Clear your mind

The Possible weight loss method demands that participants have an open mind free from the sensationalism and misinformation of the media.

You should never trust anything you read online or see on TV on diet and health unless it has been thoroughly investigated and verified. As a result, one should proceed with caution when taking them.

Believe in what you are doing

While you are implementing this method, it is crucial that you have confidence in yourself. You'll be able to alter your behaviors and become a more fit version of yourself.

Have complete faith in your new lifestyle and resist the urge to let anyone divert you from your weight loss plan. "There's no better feeling than being slender."

Eliminate negative thinking

Negative thinking violates the rules! Positive thinking is necessary to eradicate the negative ones.

Tell yourself, "I know I can successfully change my eating habits and my life," the next time you feel like giving up.

We promise you will start to feel more upbeat and confident about your efforts to embrace a new lifestyle if you repeat this sentence at least five times a day or just use it to replace any negative thoughts.

Set Goals and Positive Affirmations

Set and meet your own objectives! Choose three affirmations, such as "yes I can," "I am a disciplined body, mind, and soul," or "Being fitter is awesome," before you begin making dietary and lifestyle adjustments. These encouraging words will lift your spirits.

Build Support

Building a support network will enable you to remain committed to your objectives.

It will not only alter your way of living but also create a space where you feel comfortable discussing your successes and setbacks.

Make connections with your neighbors or coworkers who have similar objectives. Together, you may organize group workouts and discuss wholesome recipes.

Remember your Motivation

Understanding the true cause of your weight loss is similar to fueling your detox and weight reduction journey.

Consider the benefits of losing weight and the benefits of not losing weight, and write them down.

What are you prepared to give up in order to accomplish your goal?

When you realize that there are more benefits to reducing weight than there are to not losing weight, your subconscious will fully assist you in your weight loss efforts.

3

DANGERS OF LOOSING WEIGHT TOO FAST

A healthy and safe pace of weight loss is 1-2 pounds (0.45-0.9 kg) each week, according to numerous specialists.

Anything beyond that is deemed excessive weight loss and may increase your risk of several health issues, such as gallstones, muscle loss, malnourishment, and slowed metabolism.

The two most popular methods used by people to try to lose weight quickly are intense exercise and a "crash diet," which is an extremely low-calorie diet consisting of less than 800 calories per day.

Since eating a very low-calorie diet is frequently a simpler way to lose weight than exercising, people frequently choose this choice. But if you're only beginning an exercise regimen or diet, you can drop a lot more weight than 2 pounds (0.9 kg) in your first week.

Rapid weight reduction during this initial phase is rather typical. It's typical to refer to the weight you lose during this period as "water weight."

Glycogen is the energy stored in your body that is used up when you eat less calories than your body expels. Because your body's glycogen and water are linked, when you burn glycogen for energy, your body also releases water. For this reason, throughout your first week, you may see a significant decrease in weight. After your body burns through its glycogen reserves, you should lose 1-2 pounds (0.45-0.9 kg) every week on average.

Risks of Losing Weight Too Fast

Although it could seem alluring, trying to lose weight quickly is typically not advised. Rapid weight loss diets are sometimes extremely low in calories and nutrients. This could put you at danger for a number of health issues, particularly if you stick to a fast-paced diet for a long period of time.

These are some dangers associated with rapid weight loss.

You May Lose Muscle

It's not always the case that decreasing fat equals losing weight.

Even while an extremely low-calorie diet can make you lose weight quickly, a large portion of that weight might be made up of water and muscle. 25 participants in one study were given a very low-calorie diet of 500 calories per day for five weeks. They also subjected 22 participants to a 12-week low-calorie diet consisting of 1,250 calories per day.

Following the study, the researchers discovered that the weight losses in both groups were comparable. But compared to those on a low-calorie diet, individuals who followed a very low-calorie diet lost more than six times as much muscle.

It May Slow Down Your Metabolism

Your metabolism may slow down if you lose weight too quickly.

Your metabolic rate is the determinant of your daily calorie expenditure. You burn less calories each day if your metabolism is slower. According to a number of studies, cutting calories quickly can result in a daily caloric reduction of up to 23%. Loss of muscle and a decrease in hormones that control metabolism, such as thyroid hormone, are two reasons why metabolisms slow down on extremely low-calorie diets.

Regretfully, your metabolism may continue to decline for some time after you stop dieting.

It May Cause Nutritional Deficiencies

You run the danger of having a nutritional deficit if you don't consume enough calories on a daily basis.

This is due to the fact that a low-calorie diet makes it difficult to get enough of some essential nutrients like iron, folate, and vitamin B12.

Several consequences stem from insufficient dietary intake:

Hair Loss: Inadequate calorie intake can deprive the body of essential nutrients necessary for hair growth, potentially causing hair loss.

Extreme Fatigue: Low-calorie diets lacking in iron, vitamin B12, and folate may result in severe fatigue and anemia.

Weakened Immune System: Insufficient calories and nutrients can compromise immune function, heightening susceptibility to infections.

Fragile Bones: A scarcity of vitamin D, calcium, and phosphorus in one's diet might lead to weakened and brittle bones. However, adopting a diet abundant in whole, unprocessed foods can avert such nutritional deficiencies. These foods, while low in calories per gram, are satisfying and can assist in weight loss.

Gallstones: Weight loss may trigger the formation of gallstones. Reduced food intake slows the release of digestive juices from the gallbladder, potentially allowing the accumulation of substances that form gallstones. These stones can obstruct the gallbladder opening, causing severe pain and indigestion.

Additional Effects: Swift weight reduction often involves drastic calorie limitation or extreme diets, causing insufficient intake of vital nutrients such as vitamins, minerals, and protein, leading to deficiencies affecting overall health and immune function. Moreover, rapid weight loss can prompt the body to utilize muscle tissue for energy, resulting in muscle loss.

This can lower metabolism and make it harder to maintain weight loss in the long term.

Dehydration and Electrolyte Imbalance: Rapid weight loss can lead to dehydration and imbalance in electrolytes like sodium and potassium, which are essential for various bodily functions. This can cause fatigue, dizziness, and heart irregularities.

Reduced Metabolism: Severely restricting calories can signal the body to slow down metabolism to conserve energy. This can make it harder to continue losing weight or maintain weight loss in the long run.

Loss of Bone Density: In extreme cases of rapid weight loss, inadequate nutrient intake can lead to a reduction in bone density, increasing the risk of osteoporosis and fractures.

Impaired Immune Function: Inadequate nutrition can weaken the immune system, making the body more susceptible to infections and illnesses.

It's essential to aim for a gradual and sustainable rate of weight loss, typically recommended at around 1-2 pounds per week. Sustainable weight loss involves making healthier lifestyle choices, including balanced nutrition, regular physical activity, and adopting habits that can be maintained in the long term. Consulting a healthcare professional or a registered dietitian before starting any weight loss program is advisable to ensure it is safe and appropriate for individual health needs.

4

DIETERY APPROACH FOR WEIGHT LOSS

There are several dietary approaches that people consider for weight loss, each with its unique principles and methods. Here are some popular dietary approaches:

Calorie Restriction: This approach involves reducing overall calorie intake, creating a calorie deficit that leads to weight loss. It can involve portion control, tracking calories, or following specific calorie guidelines.

Low-Carb Diets: These diets, such as the ketogenic diet or Atkins diet, restrict carbohydrate intake and emphasize consuming fats and proteins. The aim is to shift the body into a state of ketosis, where it burns fat for fuel.

Low-Fat Diets: Focusing on reducing fat intake, particularly saturated fats, is a traditional approach to weight loss. It often involves choosing leaner protein sources and limiting high-fat foods.

Intermittent Fasting: This is a method that alternates between periods of eating and fasting.

Methods vary, such as the 16/8 method (fasting for 16 hours, eating within an 8-hour window) or alternate-day fasting.

Mediterranean Diet: Based on the traditional eating patterns of countries bordering the Mediterranean Sea, this diet emphasizes fruits, vegetables, whole grains, legumes, lean proteins (especially fish), and healthy fats (olive oil, nuts).

Plant-Based Diets: Vegetarian and vegan diets focus on plant-based foods, excluding or minimizing animal products. They emphasize fruits, vegetables, legumes, grains, nuts, and seeds.

Paleo Diet: This diet aims to mimic the eating patterns of our Paleolithic ancestors by focusing on whole foods, lean proteins, fruits, vegetables, nuts, and seeds while avoiding processed foods, grains, and dairy.

Whole30: This is a 30-day program that eliminates certain food groups (like sugar, alcohol, grains, legumes, and dairy) to reset eating habits and focus on whole foods.

Mindful Eating: Not a strict diet, but a practice that involves being present and attentive while eating, paying attention to hunger cues, and enjoying food without distractions, which can naturally result in better eating decisions and portion management.

DASH Diet: The Dietary Approaches to Stop Hypertension (DASH) diet emphasizes fruits, vegetables, lean proteins, whole grains, and low-fat dairy while limiting sodium intake. It's originally designed to lower blood pressure but is also beneficial for weight management.

Flexitarian Diet: This approach encourages plant-based eating while allowing occasional meat and other animal products. It focuses on adding more plant-based foods to the diet while minimizing processed and high-calorie foods.

The Zone Diet: This diet emphasizes a balance of macronutrients, particularly the ratio of carbohydrates, proteins, and fats in each meal. It focuses on keeping insulin levels in a 'zone' to promote weight loss.

The Volumetrics Diet: Developed by a nutritionist, this diet emphasizes eating low-calorie, high-volume foods like fruits, vegetables, whole grains, and lean proteins to feel full on fewer calories.

The 5:2 Diet: Involves eating normally for five days a week and significantly restricting calories (usually around 500-600 calories) for the remaining two non-consecutive days. Intermittent fasting is known to assist in weight loss.

The Blood Type Diet: This diet suggests that your blood type determines which foods are best for you. It recommends specific foods for each blood type to optimize health and manage weight.

The Alkaline Diet: This diet focuses on consuming alkaline foods (fruits, vegetables, nuts, legumes) to balance the body's pH levels. It avoids acidic foods (meat, dairy, processed foods) and aims to promote overall health and weight loss.

The Fasting-Mimicking Diet (FMD): Involves periodic fasting for a few days per month or following a specific diet pattern that mimics the effects of fasting, potentially aiding in weight loss and overall health benefits.

When considering any dietary approach for weight loss, it's important to ensure it aligns with personal health goals, preferences, and is sustainable for the long term. Consulting with a healthcare provider or a registered dietitian is beneficial to find the most suitable dietary plan for individual needs and health conditions.

5

EXERCISE PLAN

Creating an exercise plan specifically for weight loss involves a combination of cardiovascular exercises, strength training, and consistency. Here's a sample exercise plan:

Cardiovascular Exercise (3-5 days a week): Aim for 30-60 minutes of moderate-intensity cardio activities such as brisk walking, jogging, cycling, swimming, or using cardio machines at the gym.

Incorporate interval training (HIIT) 1-2 times a week for shorter, more intense bursts of exercise followed by brief rest periods.

Strength Training (2-3 days a week): Include 2-3 sessions of strength training targeting major muscle groups using bodyweight exercises, resistance bands, free weights, or weight machines.

Focus on exercises like squats, lunges, push-ups, rows, and planks. As strength increases, start with lesser weights and progressively increase resistance. **Find Activities You Enjoy:** Choosing activities you love increases the likelihood of sticking to your fitness routine. It could be hiking, dancing, playing a sport, or any activity that keeps you engaged.

Flexibility and Stretching (Regularly): Integrate flexibility exercises like yoga or dedicated stretching routines to improve flexibility, reduce muscle soreness, and enhance overall mobility.

Progressive Overload: Gradually increase the intensity, duration, or resistance of your workouts over time to continue challenging your body and promoting further weight loss.

Consistency and Rest: Plan regular exercise sessions throughout the week while allowing for rest days to prevent burnout and support muscle recovery. Consistency is Key. Establish a regular exercise routine and stick to it. Consistency over time yields better results than sporadic intense workouts.

Mindful Movement: Incorporate movement into daily activities, such as taking the stairs, walking instead of driving short distances, or incorporating short bouts of activity throughout the day.

Remember, combining this exercise plan with a balanced diet and healthy lifestyle choices is key to successful weight loss. Additionally, it's essential to start gradually and listen to your body to prevent injury and ensure long-term adherence to your exercise routine. Consulting a fitness professional or personal trainer can provide tailored guidance based on individual fitness levels and goals.

6

ADAPTIVE TACTICE

Adaptive tactics for weight loss involve flexible, personalized strategies that can be adjusted based on individual needs, challenges, and changing circumstances. These tactics focus on adapting behaviors, routines, and approaches to suit different situations and promote sustainable weight loss. Here are some adaptive tactics:

Flexible Eating Patterns: Instead of rigid diets, adopt flexible eating patterns like intuitive eating or mindful eating. Listen to your body's hunger and fullness cues, and adjust meal timings and portions accordingly.

Behavioral Awareness: Become conscious of your own eating behaviors, emotions, and triggers. Acknowledge these triggers and modify your response to effectively handle them without resorting to food as a comfort or a way to decompress.

Mindfulness Practices: Incorporate mindfulness techniques into daily routines. Implementing these practices can effectively handle stress, enhance self-awareness, and deter impulsive, emotional eating.

Consistent Adaptability: Recognize that adaptability is a key aspect of long-term success. Embrace the idea that adjustments to strategies and behaviors are a normal part of the journey and necessary for sustained progress.

Adaptive tactics for weight loss prioritize flexibility, self-awareness, and responsiveness to individual needs and circumstances. They empower individuals to navigate challenges, make informed choices, and maintain a balanced and adaptable approach to achieve and sustain their weight loss goals

7

DRINK LOTS OF WATER

While water is beneficial for weight loss, it's important to note that it's not a magic solution for significant weight reduction on its own. However, incorporating adequate hydration into a balanced diet and active lifestyle can support overall health and complement weight loss efforts.

Drinking water in the morning can also offer potential benefits, it's essential to remember that weight loss is a complex process influenced by various factors like diet, physical activity, and overall lifestyle. Drinking water alone, even if done consistently in the morning, is unlikely to lead to significant weight loss without other lifestyle changes. However, incorporating this habit as part of a comprehensive weight loss strategy that includes a balanced diet and regular exercise can contribute positively to overall health and weight management.

Drinking plenty of water can contribute to weight loss in several ways especially drinking water first thing in the morning can potentially support weight loss in a few ways:

Boosts Metabolism: Drinking water upon waking up can kickstart your metabolism. It temporarily increases your metabolic rate, which might help burn more calories throughout the day. Boosts Metabolism: Drinking water temporarily increases resting energy expenditure (metabolism). Studies suggest that drinking water can slightly boost the number of calories you burn, although this effect is modest.

Hydration: After a night's sleep, the body can be mildly dehydrated. Drinking water in the morning helps rehydrate the body, aiding in various bodily functions, including metabolism and digestion.

Curbs Appetite: Drinking water before breakfast may create a sense of fullness, leading to reduced calorie intake during the first meal of the day. This has the potential to prevent overeating and encourage better portion control.

Detoxification: Some proponents suggest that drinking water in the morning can help flush out toxins and waste products, aiding in the body's natural detoxification processes. While this claim is not fully supported by scientific evidence, proper hydration does support kidney function, which is essential for waste elimination.

Promotes Healthy Habits: Starting the day with a glass of water can set a positive tone for the rest of the day, encouraging healthy hydration habits and potentially making individuals more conscious of their overall water intake.

Appetite Control: Water can help reduce feelings of hunger. Occasionally, the body can misinterpret thirst as hunger, resulting in unnecessary snacking or overeating. Drinking water before meals can create a sense of fullness, which may result in consuming fewer calories during the meal.

Calorie-Free Hydration: Choosing water over sugary beverages reduces calorie intake. Beverages like sodas, juices, and sweetened teas can be high in calories and contribute to weight gain when consumed in excess. Water, on the other hand, is calorie-free and can help in maintaining overall calorie balance.

Supports Exercise Performance: Staying hydrated is crucial for optimal exercise performance. Proper hydration enables better endurance and stamina during workouts, allowing you to burn more calories and potentially aid in weight loss efforts.

Enhances Metabolic Processes: Water is involved in various metabolic processes, including those related to fat metabolism. Proper hydration ensures that these processes function efficiently, potentially supporting fat breakdown and utilization.

Reduces Water Retention: Paradoxically, staying hydrated can help prevent water retention by signaling to the body that it doesn't need to hold onto excess water. This can contribute to a temporary reduction in water weight.

8

PLAN AHEAD

Planning ahead can actually support weight loss rather than hinder it. Here's how:

Therefore, planning ahead is an effective strategy for weight loss. It encourages healthier eating habits, supports portion control, reduces stress, and aids in maintaining consistency—a key aspect of successful weight management.

Planning plays a crucial role in supporting weight loss by providing structure, organization, and a roadmap for achieving fitness goals. Here's how planning contributes to successful weight loss:

By incorporating planning into a weight loss journey, individuals can create a framework that supports their goals, promotes healthier habits, and increases the likelihood of long-term success. Flexibility within the plan allows for adjustments and adaptations, ensuring it remains effective and sustainable.

Healthy Food Choices: Planning meals in advance allows you to make healthier food choices. When meals are pre-planned, it's easier to opt for nutritious options rather than grabbing convenient, often less healthy, choices.

Portion Control: Planning meals and snacks ahead of time allows for better portion control. It helps prevent overeating and reduces the likelihood of consuming excessive calories.

Steering clear of impulsive eating: is more attainable when meals are pre-planned, reducing the likelihood of emotional or impulsive eating. It reduces the reliance on fast food or unhealthy snacks and encourages sticking to the planned, healthier options.

Mindful Eating: Planning meals in advance encourages mindful eating. It promotes awareness of what and how much you're consuming, fostering a healthier relationship with food.

Grocery Shopping: Planning meals in advance often involves making a grocery list. This helps in buying healthier ingredients and prevents unnecessary purchases of unhealthy foods.

Structured Approach: A well-thought-out plan provides a structured approach to weight loss. It includes strategies for diet, exercise, and lifestyle changes, helping to stay on track and avoid impulsive decisions.

Meal Preparation and Portion Control: Planning meals in advance allows for healthier food choices, portion control, and reduced reliance on fast food or unhealthy options. It ensures access to nutritious meals, preventing last-minute unhealthy eating.

Consistency: A plan encourages consistency in both diet and exercise routines. Having a set schedule for workouts and meals helps form habits and ensures regularity, which is crucial for sustainable weight loss.

Accountability and Monitoring: Planning allows for tracking progress. It enables individuals to monitor their food intake, exercise frequency, and weight changes, providing insights into what's working and what needs adjustment.

Anticipating Challenges: A good plan considers potential obstacles and challenges. It prepares individuals to face hurdles, find solutions, and avoid situations that might derail their progress.

Time Management: Planning optimizes time by scheduling workouts, meal prep, and other healthy habits. It helps in allocating time effectively for exercise and self-care amid other commitments.

Empowerment and Motivation: A well-structured plan provides a sense of control and empowerment. Seeing progress towards goals motivates individuals to continue their efforts.

Reduction of Stress: Having a plan in place reduces decision-making stress. Knowing what to eat and when to exercise removes uncertainty and reduces stress associated with choices.

Establishing Clear Goals: Planning allows individuals to set specific, achievable, and realistic weight loss goals. Having a clear target helps focus efforts and measure progress.

9

CONCLUSION

Losing weight involves a multifaceted journey that extends beyond merely shedding pounds. It encompasses a holistic approach involving dietary changes, regular physical activity, behavioral adjustments, and mental resilience.

While the ultimate goal might be losing weight, the focus should also be on improving overall health and well-being. Sustainable weight loss isn't about quick fixes or extreme measures; it's about adopting healthy habits that can be maintained for the long term.

Understanding individual needs, preferences, and health conditions is crucial. There's no one-size-fits-all approach to weight loss. It's about finding a balance that works for an individual's lifestyle, preferences, and health status.

Weight loss journeys often involve setbacks and plateaus, but these moments are opportunities for learning and growth. Consistency, patience, and a positive mindset are key elements in achieving and maintaining a healthier weight.

Ultimately, while weight loss can have significant health benefits, it's essential to celebrate progress, prioritize health over numbers, and embrace the journey towards a healthier and more fulfilling life.

Rather than lounging around wishing, seeking divine intervention for something great to occur, get it going. Individuals that are doing whatever they might want to do show up seriously fascinating. Furthermore, the seriously fascinating you are, the more appealing you'll show up. Contemplate VIPs, we watch them since they are great at what they in all actuality do on screen or in front of an audience. The equivalent for your #1 YouTube powerhouse, they appear to have invigorating lives and offer every one of the extraordinary things they love doing. Indeed, you can do those things as well! Not precisely like them, but rather in your own specific manner.

6)   Put The best version of yourself Forward:

While you will interact with others, don't leave the house not thinking often about what you resemble. Regardless of whether you're not the most appealing individual you will show up more alluring in light of the fact that you invest heavily in your general show.

7) Choose To Be Content Regardless of anything else:

In any event, while you're having a terrible day or things aren't going right, decide to be content come what may. Cheerful individuals draw in blissful individuals. You are not your conditions, accordingly whatever you're going through is emotional to what you see you're going through. Certainly, you could be going through a few truly difficult situations, nonetheless, assuming you as of now feel terrible, for what reason do whatever will exacerbate you. All things considered, pursue a choice to develop through what you go through, rather than regretting your circumstance. Since the more joyful you are the more alluring you'll show up.

Step by step instructions to Make Yourself More Appealing

1. Find the right hairdo or hair tone for you : Not every person can pull off bangs or platinum blonde hair. It could require some trial and error, and long periods of experimentation to track down your optimal hairdo.

•	Pick a hair variety that is inside a couple of shades of your normal tone so it is not difficult to keep up with, and won't look crazy once your underlying foundations fill in. To go lighter, consider adding unobtrusive features instead of another general tone.

•	Consider your face shape while tracking down the right hair style. The thought is to hype your regular highlights and try not to misrepresent the face shape. Think about the accompanying hairdo ideas: Ladies with round faces look great with deviated haircuts with a side part. Ladies with square faces ought to attempt calculated sways, long or medium-length layered cuts, or side-cleared bangs. Ladies with long, meager countenances look great with short or medium-length hair with unobtrusive waves, and ought to try not to get gruff, straight-across bangs.

Those with oval or heart-formed appearances can pull of basically any hairdo (good for them). The key is to try!

2. Keep up with your own cleanliness: Not exclusively will this work on your general appearance, it will assist with forestalling the turn of events and spread of contaminations and different sicknesses.

• Clean your teeth each day and night. This will assist with keeping your teeth white, leave you with new breath, and above all, keep your teeth and gums solid.

• Shower consistently, regardless of whether you need to wash your hair. In the event that you lack the opportunity to shower, make certain to essentially flush your face and underarms with a washcloth and cleanser.

• Shave, tweeze, wax or potentially pluck when essential. Assuming that you're going for a "whiz" or "tough" look, that is fine as well, yet do it deliberately, not out of sluggishness.

3. Tackle skincare issues: Having good expectations about your skin is critical, on the grounds that it is the main thing everyone sees when they check you out. On the off chance that you are stressed over imperfections, scars, or sunspots, converse with your dermatologist to track down the fitting treatment choices. There are different creams and balms out there to assist with blurring dull spots or scars.

• Wear sunscreen or a cap on the off chance that you anticipate being out in the sun for a lengthy timeframe. This will forestall sun related burns and dim spots, and, surprisingly, more critically, will shield your skin from the destructive impacts of sun openness.

• Hydrate. Remaining hydrated keeps your skin looking sound and brilliant, and gives you the energy you want to remain solid.

4. Get in shape: This doesn't be guaranteed to mean getting thinner; it implies anything you desire it to mean. On the off chance that you might want to drop a couple of pounds, diminish your caloric admission and integrate cardio practices into your everyday daily schedule. If you have any desire to acquire muscle, then, at that point, do opposition preparing and make certain to eat a protein-rich eating routine.

- Eat natural products, vegetables, and lean proteins. These food sources are plentiful in the nutrients and supplements your body needs, and will keep your body looking and feeling perfect.

- Keep an eye out for additional sugars. Make certain to peruse food marks and be careful with additional sugars that are added to dressings, breads, and sauces.

- Eliminate liquor. Not exclusively will this work on your skin by forestalling drying out, it will save you from consuming pointless calories.

- Join a rec center or track down an activity mate. Practicing with others will assist with keeping you roused.

5. Dress properly for your body type: No matter what the event for sure's "in" right now, putting your best self forward implies wearing garments that look great on you. Patterns travel every which way, and not every one of them are figure-complimenting.

• Flaunt your best resources, and conceal your most exceedingly terrible ones. For instance, assuming you have an hourglass figure, wear perfectly sized dresses that hotshot your bends and keep away from massive or square shaped garments.

• Overlook the size on the name. Numerous ladies make a special effort to fit into some pants that are excessively little for them out of dread of "going up a size." as a general rule, how you thoroughly search in the garments matters more than the number on the tag. In addition, no one has to understand what size your jeans are!

CHAPTER TWO

Exceptionally appraised approaches to Attracting Others

1 Grin:

Continually frowning makes you look scary, serious, and exhausting. Why bother with looking wonderful assuming that everyone fears conversing with you?

2 Make yourself look agreeable: If you have any desire to draw in others, you should put yourself out there. Make an effort not to fold your arms, stay away from eye to eye connection or stand toward the side of the room. These are signs that you would rather not be irritated.

3 Be confident:

Even supermodels have uncertainties. The key is to have a comical inclination about your flaws, and not let them drag you down. Regardless of whether you trust it, start letting yourself know you are lovely, and that you look perfect. In the long run, you will fool yourself into really trusting it.

4 Have a comical inclination: Everyone needs to associate with individuals who make them snicker. This doesn't be guaranteed to mean telling wisecracks at regular intervals; in any event, being able to snicker at other people groups' jokes shows that you are a cheerful, carefree individual.

Dominating Excellence Tips For Women

1 Track down the right groundwork: In the event that your skin is on the shinier side, pick a cosmetics with a matte completion, or utilize a powder. In the event that your skin will in general be dry, pick a fluid establishment.

• While testing establishment tones, be certain that you are in a sufficiently bright region, utilizing regular light if conceivable. Test maybe a couple tones on your facial structure, delicately focusing on the establishment. Utilize a hand mirror to figure out which tone is ideal. The ideal tone ought to mix equally into your skin so you can never again see it.

• Ask a partner at the cosmetics counter to assist coordinate you with the right tone assuming that you are experiencing difficulty doing it without anyone else's help.

2 Utilize a concealer on trouble spots: Having an even composition will make you look more youthful and more alluring. Instances of pain points incorporate dull under-eye rings, flaws, scars, and additionally dim spots.

• Your concealer ought to be a shade or two lighter than your general establishment, and of a thicker consistency.

3 Track down an unpretentious, ordinary cosmetics schedule: The key is to improve your excellence without looking like you've heaped on cosmetics. Pick a normal that main requires a couple of moments so you can do it consistently. Utilize the accompanying rules to accomplish a characteristic, brilliant face:

•	Saturate your skin. This will assist with setting the cosmetics and eliminate any dryness.

•	Apply generally establishment and concealer, if important.

•	Wear mascara. Regardless of whether you wear no other cosmetics, a bit of mascara will immediately upgrade your eyes and make you look more female.

•	Add some pink. Shades of pink match all complexions, since we as a whole have a little regular pink in our skin. Applying an unpretentious blush to your cheeks will give you a warm, sun-kissed shine.

•	Apply an unobtrusive lip tone. Pick a variety that is one to two shades further than your regular lip tone.

CHAPTER THREE

19 Methods for being More Alluring, As indicated by Science

Alright, here's reality: Not all men are brought into the world with great looks and appeal. Bunches of folks are brought into the world with not one or the other, as a matter of fact. However, does that mean you're destined to go through your time on earth alone in your loft, with just Netflix and your canine to stay with you? By no means.

Truly while looks really do make a difference to people the same, it's a long way from the main thing with regards to tracking down an accomplice. The study of physical allure is a perplexing one that includes numerous variables, from the manner in which you smell to the state of your jaw to even the shade of the shirt you're wearing.

There are still a lot of ways of making yourself more alluring. The following are 19 methodologies to draw in the accomplice of your fantasies, whether in the club, in the recreation area, or on a hookup or dating application.

1) Make her giggle.

Everybody needs an accomplice who gets their comical inclination. In the event that you're the "entertaining person" among your companions, incline toward it. Indeed, even science says you ought to: A recent report distributed in Development and Human Conduct asked members the amount they esteem their accomplice's capacity to make them chuckle, and the outcomes, of course, uncovered that ladies genuinely care about their accomplice's humor. On the off chance that you're ready to make them chuckle, it's an incredibly alluring quality.

2) Wear shades.

Shades make folks more sultry, and there's confirmation to back it up. Master made sense of that shades make a man look strange: "The eyes are a particularly enormous wellspring of data — and weakness — for the person." Not having that data makes ladies attracted to you. They need to look further into the man behind the glasses.

3) Be great.

Turns out decent folks don't complete last. A recent report reviewed 800 individuals trying to more readily figure out the connection between philanthropy, fascination, and sex. The specialists got some information about their sexual history along with how frequently they participate in magnanimous demonstrations, for example, noble cause work and giving blood.

It just so happens, people who do beneficial things for, indeed, being great, got laid more. Additionally, while the review didn't investigate this, we'd wager that benevolent individuals are likewise magnanimous sweethearts, placing their accomplices' necessities into thought, and that is appealing.

4) Wear cologne.

Ladies find wearing cologne or a mark splash appealing, yet not for the explanation you think. It doesn't have to do with pheromones or normal smells, essentially as per a paper distributed in the Global Diary of Restorative Science. In the review, the members who were given a shower of cologne self-detailed higher certainty and said they felt more alluring.

Be that as it may, the discoveries don't end there: When a gathering of ladies were shown a quiet video of the men wearing the shower, they evaluated them hotter than the folks who weren't wearing any cologne. This implies that when you feel hotter and more certain, ladies get on that, and think that you are more appealing. (Additionally, there's the advantage of really smelling pleasant rather than like your duffel bag.)

5) Eat more garlic.

Garlic? That's right, garlic. We're a little distrustful, yet a recent report distributed in the scholastic diary Craving found that men who eat garlic smell more "wonderful" and "alluring" than the people who don't. The review proposes that eating garlic some way or another effects our stench.

To explain, having a garlic-y inhale is as yet gross, yet consuming garlic can help you a level on the alluring scale.

6) Travel with an escort.

In the event that you're gone making the rounds, get a couple of mates to be your partners. As per a review from the College of California at San Diego, individuals were evaluated as better-looking when they were in bunch photographs than in independent shots.

Credit it to something many refer to as the "team promoter impact." Individuals show up additional alluring in bunches since survey faces together makes them seem to be the gathering normal —

which can help "level out" any one individual's ugly quirks. (This doesn't, be that as it may, apply to dating applications, where you ought to never utilize a gathering photograph.)

7) Get to know a child.

However going with a company is never a terrible move, your best partner may really be a child. As indicated by research, men who got along with children were multiple times as prone to score a lady's telephone number than folks who overlooked the babies. As a matter of fact, 40% of women surrendered their digits after they saw men grinning, cooing, and conversing with the kids.

So in the event that you have a niece or nephew you're obsessed with, volunteer to watch on occasion. Their folks will probably see the value in the assistance, so it's a shared benefit for everybody.

8) Walk your canine.

Man's Dearest companion, for sure: As indicated by study, ladies were multiple times as prone to give out their telephone numbers to a person in the city on the off chance that he moved toward them with a canine than if he asked alone. Canines can assist with lubing social association, adding that canines support impression of generosity, care, and awareness.

9) Offer your razor a reprieve.

Ladies tracked down folks with weighty stubble — around 10 days' worth — to be more attractive than those with a lighter shadow, a full facial hair growth, or a totally clean-cut face. This likewise applies to gay men, who find unshaven men more appealing than clean-cut folks.

10) Expert your walk.

Nothing is a higher priority than certainty while endeavoring to draw in an accomplice, and one of the most straightforward ways of measuring a man's certainty to see how they stroll down the road.

Planned accomplices "take a gander at your clothing and second at how you walk." An Aide During Romance and Dating. "Time is on sure people's side, but instead there's a difference among meandering and walking progressively with reason.

Continuously stroll as though you understand what you're doing and where you're going."

11) Specialty your dating application profile carefully.

Individuals who utilized positive words like "imaginative," "aggressive," or "giggle" in their web based dating profiles got 33% more messages, as per a study from dating website. Referencing side interest related words like "book" or "read" — or including data about running, running, or lifting loads — gave a critical message support, as well.

Simply be cautious you're not coming on major areas of strength for excessively. Men whose first message contained words like "supper" or "beverages" saw their reaction rate plunge by 35%.

At any rate, simply ensure you have something in your Kindling, Blunder, Pivot, or Grindr profile. Preferably, that something ought to be extraordinary to you. "I feel that people should be express." "People are genuinely stressed over not wandering in light of what is considered customary, [but] I envision that people are truly giving a gigantic unfair arrangement to themselves since they aren't standing separated from the other hundred people in their geographic compass who match their age and direction models."

12) Avoid selfies.

Folks who posted selfies on their web based dating profiles got less messages. Ladies track down shirtless selfies "exceptionally ugly. Everyone needs to know someone's fit and has a pleasant body, yet you can tell that through seeing someone in dress." All things considered, have a companion snap a photograph of you, and head outside in the meantime. Men with an outside shot gathered 19% more messages, as per research.

All things considered, the "no shirtless selfies!" rule doesn't appear to hold tight gay dating applications: an examination, found that by far most of the clients display their bodies and genuine health on the application, which didn't particularly impact their chances to find a hookup.

13) Grin (be that as it may, as, gradually).

Men who let their grins spread gradually across their countenances were decided as more alluring than the individuals who put on a fast smile. The sluggish grinning folks were additionally evaluated as more dependable, showing that their demeanors may be seen as more veritable.

Blazing a smile is likewise significant while assembling an internet dating profile. "I know 14% of individuals will undoubtedly be swiped right on accepting they are smiling since evybody realizes that smiling gives thoughtfulness and congeniality." "You would rather not appear as though you're scowling, regardless of what might be shown in promotions."

14) Remain solid, yet all the same not excessively solid.

An investigation discovered that ladies evaluated "constructed" men as more physically attractive than meager, non-ripped "thin" folks and heavier, more-built "muscular" fellows. The specialists say it's similar to the Goldilocks impact: Ladies like a few muscles, yet entirely not too much. This isn't, nonetheless, the case on gay dating applications, where men evaluated a strong body as the most alluring quality in men.

15) Display your fight scars.

Ladies evaluated men with gentle scarring on their countenances as more appealing for transient indulgences than flawless folks, study found.

Females could see scars as an indication of increased manliness, the specialists accept. That is particularly evident assuming the imprints were a consequence of an injury of some sort, since that can publicize great qualities or a solid resistant framework.

16) Convey a guitar.

As indicated by a review, ladies were multiple times as prone to give a person her telephone number when he requested it while holding a guitar case than when he conveyed a games pack. Hatchet men are by and large considered "cool" and "tomfoolery." Besides, melodic capacity could likewise flag higher insight and great qualities — two characteristics essential to ladies while picking an accomplice.

17) Trench the cliché pickup line.

As per a review, individuals are bound to lean toward an individual for a drawn out relationship on the off chance that he utilizes direct opening lines ("I saw you across the room and needed to meet you. What's your name?") or on the other hand safe ones ("Do you have the open door?")

rather than pretentious come-ons ("Will we talk or continue to be a bother from a distance?").

Cocky expressions likewise cause men to appear to be less savvy and less dependable, concentrate on found.

18) Manspreading can be something to be thankful for.

Ladies evaluated men who sat with an open body pose — legs spread, arms loosened up — and utilized hand motions as more sweltering than folks who sat with their legs together and arms collapsed, scientists found. Open non-verbal communication is viewed as a sign of predominance.

Simply ensure you're remaining minimized on the off chance that you're on a jam-packed metro train.

19) Purchase a bouquet.

Just being in a room with a couple of containers of blossoms can impact the manner in which a lady sees you. At the point when blossoms were close by, women made a decision about men as hotter and more appealing than they did when the room was unfilled. Blossoms can flag sentiment and improve her temperament, the analysts say, which might help her view you all the more well.

CHAPTER FOUR

15 Principles to Build Fascination

The Absolute Most Alluring Attribute

What turns you on? Eyes? Humor? Legs?

Concentrate on shows that an individual's most alluring quality is their accessibility. Certainty is an or more, as well, however accessibility wins, without a doubt.

Fascination Tip 1: Utilize Open Non-verbal communication

Is it true or not that you are shutting yourself off to other people? We could close our non-verbal communication and appear to be inaccessible without acknowledging it:

- crossed arms

- grasping a wine glass before our stomach

- checking a telephone before our chest

- embracing a handbag to our middle

We close our non-verbal communication when we are feeling intellectually shut off, and individuals can see this a pretty far.

To look more alluring, you don't need to change your looks — you basically need to change your non-verbal communication to be more open. Non-verbal communication research has shown that keeping your middle, chest, and mid-region open to the world is the most ideal way to show accessibility.

Open non-verbal communication is more alluring than any outfit, haircut, or dance move.

Female and male non-verbal communication likewise vary. Here is an outline of female non-verbal communication to keep an eye out for:

A fascinating tale about how open non-verbal communication and liberality remain closely connected: I was people-watching at a systems administration occasion, and watched a man and lady talking. Toward the start of the discussion, the lady was holding her handbag before her chest, and the man was holding his wine glass before him. At a certain point, the man made a joke, and the two of them started to chuckle. You could see them sincerely unwind and open up. At that point, the lady swung her tote behind her and opened up her non-verbal communication. In the exceptionally one second from now, the man put his glass on the mixed drink table close to them and took out a business card. They kept talking the remainder of the evening.

*If you have any desire to add sexuality to your engaging quality you can likewise uncover your neck (think Marilyn Monroe shifting her head back and giggling).

From a non-verbal communication point of view, an open, uncovered, or stroked neck isn't just more sexy yet additionally delivers enticing pheromones. See more about this in the video above.

Financial sway (and Cup)

Handbag and cup conduct is a typical type of hindering, as well. It is the means by which somebody cooperates with their current circumstance, in light of their feelings.

For instance, in the event that a lady is feeling awkward or not drawn to somebody, she will either grip her sack firmly or place it before or covering her body. At the point when a lady is drawn in, she in a real sense and metaphorically believes that nothing should hold up traffic among her and her darling.

All kinds of people will likewise do likewise with their drinking cup, involving it as a boundary to shut out others.

On the off chance that she freely holds her satchel, and it isn't obstructing her front, this shows she is quiet and feels more fascination. Even better, on the off chance that she puts it on the floor, on a close by table, or on the rear of the seat, she needs it far removed for her connections with you.*

*If it's not too much trouble, note setting here: in the event that you are in an exceptionally open or possibly perilous area, she could be grasping her satchel for wellbeing concerns, however in a relaxed put or out on the town, this can be a decent marker.

I was really at a singles occasion an evening or two ago and watched a man and lady talking. The lady had her handbag to some degree obstructing her body and was holding the handle firmly under her arm. Then, at that point, the man told her he was a specialist, and the lady in a real sense swung her handbag over-top her shoulder, far removed. It was astounding.

Fascination Tip 2: Fronting

Fronting, or settling, is the point at which you square up your body so you are straightforwardly confronting an individual. At the point when you front somebody, you are flagging fascination and interest. According to it, "I'm here, and you are the focal point of my consideration."

At the point when you front somebody, they are the focal point of your universe.

While fronting, remember the 3 Ts:

- Toes

- Torso

- Top (or head)

Ace Tip: Here and there, you can't front. Perhaps you're situated close to one another or in a packed scene where your middles are confronting a similar course. Assuming that is the situation, read on to figure out how to show accessibility and receptiveness without fronting...

Fascination Tip 3: Pick The Right Seat At Supper

Picture this: You have a supper date coming up. Let's assume you're going to Chipotle, Olive Nursery, or the Ritz (very surprising price tags, I know).

You're with your accomplice, and there's a table before you. They sit on one of the seats. Where do you sit for ideal fascination?

1.   Seat A

2.   Seat B

3.   Seat C

4.   None of the abovementioned

Fascination Tip 4: Incline In to Show Commitment

Inclining in the direction of somebody is a nonverbal approach to letting them know you are locked in. This functions admirably in the event that you are in a gathering, and you are keen on one individual in the gathering. This will subliminally "pull" them toward you and nonverbally say, "I like you the most!"

Ace Tip: Are there items like a seat or work area in the manner? Move yourself or move the items so you can incline forward without the messiness.

Fascination Tip 5: Eye Staring

Eye staring is the strong, close demonstration of gazing at someone for an extensive stretch of time. At the point when they gaze back at you, oxytocin, or the "affection chemical," increments.

In a review, irregular outsiders were approached to gaze into one another's eyes for 2 minutes without looking away. They detailed "expanded sensations of enthusiastic love for one another."

Eye stare is strong to such an extent that it doesn't just work in people — it works with canines, as well. In another review, canines were prepared to look into their proprietors' eyes. Subsequent to getting those looks, both the proprietor and the canine had raised oxytocin levels.

Cool, isn't that so? Eye stare works for expanding fascination since oxytocin is in a real sense created in the heart.

At the point when your body discharges oxytocin, you in a real sense feel it in the heart.

Master Tip: Anything you do, don't gaze Excessively. A closeness balance model by Argyle and Senior member says assuming you gaze excessively, the other individual will look less. The most loved procedure I involved back in my school days is to visually engage, hold the contact for 3 seconds, then offer a wink and look while grinning. During a discussion, the ideal measure of eye to eye connection is between 60-70% of the time. You might actually visually connect while you're talking and more while tuning in.

Fascination Tip 6: The Pause And-Grin

You could have heard that grinning is something worth being thankful for. Furthermore, it is! I grin constantly on the grounds that I'm truly cheerful and intrigued to meet new individuals. Nonetheless, you CAN get out of hand. There's a range of grinning that you ought to attempt to remain in. I call this the Grin o-meter.

On a size of 1-10, how often do you grin in a discussion? My perfect balance for grinning is a 7. Research shows that individuals who grin all the more frequently have less status and less power1.

Betas will generally grin. Alphas don't really.

You for the most part need to grin more than not, however there's a stunt to the Grin o-meter. Utilize the pause and-grin approach:

•   Hold on until you've been presented in a discussion or are presenting yourself prior to grinning.

•   Then, as you shake your colleague's hand and say their name, grin comprehensively, as though hearing their name carried a grin to your face.

Along these lines, others will feel as though their name was so interesting to you that it made you grin splendidly. Others will "get" your joy and bliss, causing a veritable gradually expanding influence of fascination.

Activity Step: Where is your grin on the Grin o-meter? In your next discussion, rate yourself out of 10. Attempt to increment or reduction to make it an ideal 7.

Fascination Tip 7: Utilize a Careful Style

Stand by, hold up... Would you say you are anticipating doing this multitude of signals? There's a stunt to doing them...

to amplify your fascination...

furthermore, that is... to do them... slowly.

In a review, scientists found that it's great to utilize a watchful style of nonverbals when you initially meet another person. What's the significance here? Cautiousness implies:

•   utilizing more modest signals with additional exact developments

•   utilizing more slow talking rate and developments

•   inclining in reverse rather than forward

As such, relax.

This could try and conflict with some non-verbal communication signs you've advanced up to this point. Notwithstanding, think about it like the "testing stage" of a relationship. At the point when you initially meet somebody, you're an alien to them. So you would rather not fall off serious areas of strength for excessively.

After enough affinity is developed, and you begin to settle in, more forward and coordinate fascination prompts can be utilized. You'll see, when now is the right time to increase the closeness, on the off chance that their non-verbal communication begins to open up.

Fascination Tip 8: Don't Look for

How frequently have you been at a major get-together, and you've seen two or three individuals waiting around this way?

Method for being a state of mind executioner! Looking out toward the group isn't really something terrible, however it conveys your advantage lies somewhere else (otherwise known as not with yourself). Flagging this way shows to others that you're effectively NOT having a good time or engaging yourself.

All things being equal, suppose you saw 2 individuals like this:

Which gathering seems to be the one you'd need to join? I'd require the second one instantly. So to actually easily draw in individuals to you, you must carry the amusing to yourself.

•	Be locked in. Regardless of where you are, be genuinely drawn in with whomever you're with. Have a fabulous time. Tell a wisecrack. Other people who notice you might need to jump in and let loose, as well!

•	Engage yourself. Alone? No problem! You can engage yourself by communicating with whoever's close by — the barkeep, the staff, even arbitrary outsiders. Or then again, you might pull up your telephone and track down what's fascinating to you. I've two or three discussions start along these lines, where I was basically perusing my telephone, and individuals needed to know why I was giggling to such an extent.

Fascination Tip 9: Reflecting Non-verbal communication

Reflecting is the point at which you inconspicuously duplicate the non-verbal communication of the other individual. The agreement is that reflecting is H.O.T.

In one review, men evaluated a lady all the more visually captivating on the off chance that she had copied his verbal and nonverbal way of behaving during speed dating2. We will generally subliminally reflect individuals assuming we like them. The way to reflecting is being unpretentious — clear reflecting can really break affinity and lessening fascination.

Assuming somebody rests back on the wall, recline, as well. Assuming that they set up their leg, do that too.

Fascination Tip 10: Have Consistent Looks

What does your face resemble while it's resting? Tragically, mine is the exemplary resting bitch face (RBF). Others could have a "clear gaze" that seems as though they're watching paint dry. In any case, simply suppose somebody's checking out the room, prepared and eager to converse with another person, and they see this:

Look inquisitive and inspired by the climate, score to the music, be idealistic, and grin — these little signals will go quite far to turning out to be more agreeable. However, it's not so straightforward as changing your look. You must be harmonious.

What is harmoniousness? More or less, coinciding is being a similar all around. Allow me to make sense of this significant however basic idea with shapes. To begin with, you understand what a circle is. Furthermore, you understand what a triangle is. Yet, in the event that a circle attempts to turn into a triangle...

To be more appealing, your non-verbal communication and looks should be consistent.

For instance, in the event that you go up to a young lady and give her an eyebrow blaze and grin, yet you're perspiring lavishly from apprehension, and your feet are highlighted the exit since you're dreadful apprehensive... you're absolutely incongruent!

We have inside radars that go off at whatever point we're around incongruent individuals:

•   the "troublemaker" who attempts to act sure yet just puts on a show of being coldhearted and overcompensating

•   the young lady who attempts to act well known yet where it counts, she's truly uncertain and unconfident

•   the companion who attempts to act decent however is really poisonous and can't stand you

Speaking the truth about your nervousness is greatly improved. So on the off chance that your face is simply bleh, acknowledge yourself, and you'll put on a show of being more certified and amiable. Trust me — I've been in the circumstance where I've attempted to counterfeit my certainty. It won't ever work.

Activity Step: Who are you attempting to depict? Individuals can track down incongruency a pretty far. Continuously attempt to behave such as yourself, and don't expect to be an "ideal" rendition of yourself. Whenever you're out, attempt to communicate the feelings that you really feel.

Fascination Tip 11: The 5 out of 15 Rule

The 5 out of 15 rule of being a tease is to contact somebody multiple times in 15 minutes or less. The touch can be the point at which you first methodology somebody, and you can sprinkle contacts to a great extent when you make a joke or offer chuckling. Pick your area of touch:

• The arm. This is a protected spot that I like to begin with. The upper arm is the most secure; going nearer to the hand draws nearer to closeness.

- The shoulder is a more weak region since it's nearer to the neck, however can be utilized on the off chance that it's a speedy tap. Contacting here is best saved for assuming that you've areas of strength for fabricated.

- The body. Stay away from the body except if you're prepared to increase the closeness.

The 5 out of 15 rule is incredible in light of the fact that surprising touch discharges small dosages of dopamine.

Contact is important to the point that even individuals from the most reduced standing in India were called untouchables. Unforeseen touch is surprisingly better since it really makes our pulse increment.

Utilize startling contacts to build excitement and fervor all through your discussion.

Genius Tip: Measure your touch. You would rather not touch somebody who isn't inviting it. Ladies showed contact from an outsider is the best intrusion of protection, while men felt the equivalent when it came from another man. On the off chance that their non-verbal communication is loose and open and quickly closes after your touch, then, at that point, it's a decent sign your touch is excluded.

Fascination Tip 12: The Right Side

Did you had any idea there is a favored side we like individuals to be on? It's either our left half of our body or our right side. Assuming that individuals are on my Off-base side, I feel more abnormal and clumsier than expected.

For what reason do we have a "liked" side? The OLD hypothesis states:

- Handshake goes about as an anchor.

- At the point when we shake hands, we make oblivious positive feelings, and ordinarily, we are on the individual's right side when we shake hands.

- Remaining on this side reproduces these feelings unwittingly.

At the point when an individual tells the truth and helpful, stand to one side to fabricate entrust with them. At the point when somebody is shutting down or being dishonest, stand to one side to break compatibility and make pressure and stress.

Activity Step: Do you see an individual acting stranger or more shaky than expected while you're remaining on one side? Have a go at exchanging over to the opposite side. Use changes to make it more subtle:

- Get a napkin or drink.

- Go to the restroom.

- Taste some water.

Assuming they begin livening straight up, that is a decent sign you're on their right side. Test each side for 30 seconds to 2 minutes, then, at that point, test once more to affirm their right side.

You might ask your accomplices or companions their seat inclinations the following time you hang out at a café or the films. Move from one side to the next, and check whether you notice apprehensive or tense motions.

Their Feet Like You

The feet act as an immediate impression of an individual's mentality. The key is seeing where a person's feet are pointed.

At the point when the feet are pointed straightforwardly toward someone else, this is an indication of fascination, or at any rate, real premium. If, then again, the feet are pointed away or toward the leave, that is an indication that fascination is most likely not there.

Here is the reality: Fascination isn't just about looks. You become more appealing when you attract individuals with your character and your mystique. Appealing nonverbals help a great deal too! Make certain to utilize these signs to be more alluring to everybody you meet.

Fascination Tip 13: Asserting Space

An incredible method for building your certainty and fascination is to occupy room. Envision the most alluring individual in the room — would they say they are logical concealing in the corner, nestled into a ball? Presumably not.

The alluring and certain individual is extensive. They're enormous. Furthermore, they take up a ton of visual space. Have a go at extending yourself:

• Lay your arms on the armrests.

• Enlarge your legs.

• Put your effects on objects to "guarantee them."

You can likewise coordinate space through your current circumstance by the method of continue to move. Think in your past to one of the longest, funnest days you've at any point had. For my purposes, that was the point at which I went on a new outing to the ocean side with Sienna and my better half to another ocean side house! What's more, chances are, your experience likewise includes oddity and various encounters.

What's more, here's where continuing to move becomes possibly the most important factor...

Various conditions make unique, novel encounters.

For instance, have you at any point been on an espresso date or conference, and it appeared to keep going for quite a long time? This is definitely not a terrible sign, however you probably recall it as one unmistakable experience.

Presently balance that with one more date where you move to 3 spots:

- To begin with, you start in the workplace.

- Then, at that point, you move to a bistro.

- A short time later, you carry your accomplice to a pastry bistro.

Notice how in every one of the 3 distinct areas, you can welcome new sentiments and feelings.

Maybe you could have even seen that vehicle sellers do this a ton. They meet you at an open parcel to examine the highlights of a vehicle.

Then, at that point, take you to the anteroom to stand by before the test drive. Then to the workplace, then to the vehicle once more. This provides you with the sensation of considering buying for a long time1.

This works in business, yet additionally in making personal connections, too. Singles on dates ought to do this to "feel" like they've known one another more drawn out than they really do.

Activity Step: Before your next large date or conference, plan out 3 unique areas you can move to. Turn to new areas on the off chance that there's a respite in discussion, or you need to move to a spic and span subject of discussion. Keep them alert and aware. Continue to move!

Fascination Tip 14: Motion With Your Hands

We love to see individuals' hands. Investigations have discovered that when we can't see individuals' hands, we experience difficulty confiding in them. At the point when you put your hands in your pockets, fold them under the table, or conceal them behind a coat, your engaging quality declines since you're immediately making cautioning signs to other people.

All things being equal, consistently have your hands appearing. Concentrates on show the best motions to use in dating circumstances are sweeping ones. These motions increment your apparent receptiveness and even strength, at times.

Activity Step: Need to realize the best hand motions you can utilize at the present time? Head on over to the rundown of best hand motions you ought to be aware.

Fascination Tip 15: Quit Being Exhausting

Our minds resemble truly hungry little children. They are effectively exhausted and they request to be taken care of with engaging chunks. Being "hot" basically isn't sufficient.

New York Times top of the line creator and formative sub-atomic researcher John Medina found that the mind has an exceptionally limited capacity to focus. Our minds are drawn to individuals and things that are charming, intriguing, and locking in. Fortunately, you are a captivating, fascinating, and drawing face to face!

It's appealing to intrigue.

Indeed, I have met large number of individuals at talking occasions, gatherings, and systems administration parties — and I have never met a solitary exhausting individual.

At times we act exhausting in light of the fact that we fear being viewed as "abnormal" or "unique." So we have a similar brain numbingly wearing social contents out:

- "What do you do?"

- "Where are you from?"

- "How's the climate?"

We don't share how we truly feel, we conceal our peculiarities, and we attempt to fit in. However, guess what? Fitting in sucks! It's dull and ugly.

Our apprehension about not fitting in makes us exhausting.

Logical exploration has shown us that there are devices we can use to battle the exhausting, increment our allure, and make us more vital. How would we do this? We figure out how to intrigue.

The most effective method to Be Moved toward in a Bar

Have you at any point been at a bar and remained there endlessly standing by some more? Truth be told, your non-verbal communication probably won't convey transparency. Rather than shutting individuals out, attempt to dismiss your middle from the bar and toward the focal point of the room or where the greater part of individuals are.

Keep in mind, you additionally need to abstain from looking for ways of behaving, so don't go scanning the space for somebody to come approach you. Appear as though you're having a great time, regardless of whether you're isolated!

CHAPTER FIVE

The most effective method to Be Alluring As a Man

How would you rate your own engaging quality as a man? Here are a few hints to expand your fascination:

1: Look Savvy

A distant memory are the times of seeming as though you just returned from a conflict with lions. Or then again seeming to be Rambo.

In a review of 5,500 singles somewhere in the range of 21 and 76, an incredible 63% of individuals said a messy appearance was their greatest relationship big issue. Before taking into account moving toward anybody, you must be prepped and ready:

• Get new breath. Need to know quite possibly of MY greatest side road? A horrendous instance of halitosis. Try to brush your tongue prior to going out, and consistently two or three mints in your back pocket. A few mints with sugars leave your mouth significantly stinkier a short time later, so try to put resources into quality tablets.

• Clean those fingernails. Check your nails at this moment. Do you nibble them? Is there gunk from the previous evening's mud wrestling match? How do your fingernail skin look? You may not mind, yet others may. Consider utilizing a nail document to manage those harsh nails, and consider moving beyond the vice of nail gnawing.

• Prep your garments. You don't need to get ready, however in the event that you're dressing to dazzle, it very well may be smart to press your shirt, clean your shoes (child wipes make all the difference!), and utilize a build up roller to dispose of those irregular bits of build up.

• Style your hair. Contingent upon your hair, you can smooth it back for a spotless/proficient look, or add a gel to give it some volume and surface. What's more, indeed, it is an unquestionable necessity to wash your hair.

2: Be The Focal point of Consideration

While moving toward a gathering, how would you move toward them?

1. directly, sure and guaranteed

2. skittishly, apprehensive and abnormal

3. not by any means

You could think a) is the most intelligent response, and you're correct! In any case, there's a proviso...

Drawing closer straightforwardly may not be the most ideal decision. This is an error men frequently make.

Why? Since you're in a real sense setting yourself in opposition to them.

All things being equal, go inside the gathering (by requesting a beverage and pivoting, pardoning yourself in, and so on), and be in the middle1. This gets 2 things done:

1.   You'll seem to be a pioneer and show up with others, not against them.

2.   Other individuals who see you in a bar will view you as having expanded esteem.

Going inside the gathering takes a ton of boldness, so in the event that you don't have the certainty to do that yet, no problem! Gradually move gradually up, and at some point, you will arrive.

3: Directing Touch

You can put a hand on the little of your accomplice's back, simply over the jeans, on the off chance that they are your heartfelt interest. You can utilize the directing touch for however long you are pushing toward an entryway. Hold your hand on the little of their back for as long as 7 seconds, and utilize a strong/firm strain — a similar tension you'd use to push a shopping cart1.

Ace Tip: Utilize the directing touch sparingly, and don't utilize it at least a few times in a brief timeframe.

4: Utilize Quiet Aromas

Which aromas are ladies drawn to the most? The smell of experience, pine trees, and masculine sweat? Reconsider. As indicated by research, ladies are really drawn to child powder and cucumber. Sadly, you may be somewhat bizarre hefting around a cucumber. Notwithstanding, child powder can be utilized as an incredible underarm antiperspirant!

The most effective method to Be Alluring As a Lady

To be appealing as a lady, you must convey the right messages. Here are a few signs you can use for your potential benefit:

1: Wear Heels

All kinds of people love heels (albeit, here and there we don't very much want to wear them!).

Individuals love the vibe of them and the hard "clicking" sound they make when you stroll on hard ground surface. Wearing heels makes the deception of level while angling the back, extending the legs, and further developing stance. Likewise, heels add swing to a lady's step by fortifying the center and pelvic floor.

2: The Push-Pull

While you're messed near and living it up, don't go in for the play hit. I see this one a great deal, particularly in youngsters. A few ladies even hit hard, however this is a moment compatibility breaker for some individuals since it signals hostility.

All things considered, get their arm and push them away, gradually delivering their arm. The push-pull ought to last at least 3 seconds. It's an extraordinary method for building your touch association without harming them. Nonetheless, the push-pull can likewise be compatibility breaking, contingent upon the circumstance, particularly on the off chance that you haven't grown sufficient affinity yet.

3: Streak The Merchandise

Actually no, not those merchandise! There is a significantly more unobtrusive approach to flagging fascination: the palms and wrist. To increase fascination and gentility, ensure your palms and wrists are uncovered. Numerous ladies select the limp wrist prompt, which signals accommodation and a readiness to be overwhelmed.

4: Utilize Yummy Fragrances

Do you involve fragrances in your fascination arsenal? As indicated by research, there are explicit aromas that men are drawn to. Men had the most elevated excitement increment of 40% when they smelled pumpkin pie joined with a lavender fragrance. Cinnamon additionally functions admirably. In any case, fragrance doesn't function admirably, with the most elevated of just a 3% increment.

Activity Step: To expand this, have a go at applying a characteristic lavender oil to your wrists and neck region. Stock up your vehicle and handbag with pumpkin pie deodorizers, and request any pastries that have cinnamon, for greatest adequacy.

5: Flushed and Blushed

At the point when we are drawn to somebody, blood will stream to our face, making our cheeks get red. This ends up copying the climax impact where we get flushed. It is a developmental way the body attempts to draw in the other gender. The reason why ladies wear blush. This blood stream likewise occurs with lips and eyes. The redder the lips and the more white the eyes, the more prolific and alluring somebody is.

Activity Step: Wear red lipstick. Red is the variety that has been displayed to draw in the most solicitations.

Noticing that: Whoever you are, somebody will adore you is significant.

So assuming that you've done everything expressed in this book:

- You've chipped away at your methodology.

- You've nailed your alluring non-verbal communication.

- You've dominated your interactive abilities.

Be patient, and act naturally!

It's simply an issue of tracking down the ideal individual, not the vast majority!

Figure out The Code on Looks

The human face is continually conveying messages, and we use it to comprehend the individual's goals when we address them.

In Unravel, we plunge profound into these miniature articulations to show you how to in a flash get on them and comprehend the importance behind what is shared with you.

CHAPTER SIX

12 Methods for causing YOURSELF LOOK AND To feel MORE Appealing, As per SCIENCE

A basic change in outlook can make you see yourself in an entirely different light. Assuming you're having a down outlook on your appearance, you can simplify changes that don't have anything to do with weight reduction.

• Research proposes being thoughtful to other people and having intercourse can support how you feel about your looks.

• Specialists likewise propose embracing humor and fixing your stance can likewise assist with certainty.

Get your perspiration on.

Start to perspire and it could assist with cheering you up.

You could fear practice however it can play a major figure assisting yourself with feeling more appealing.

We're not simply discussing activity's impact on your body truly — practice is an incredible method for carving out opportunity to get out your hostility, possess some energy for yourself, and delivery endorphins, a compound that can work on your mind-set. A recent report by the College of Turku found that individuals who practiced revealed an expansion in certainty.

"Practice is an extraordinary method for feeling more alluring," April Masini, a relationship and manners master, told INSIDER. "In addition to the fact that you are providing yourself with an endowment of wellness, yet you're delivering endorphins and adjusting work, play and taking care of oneself."

Offer a few commendations.

Let those close to you know how phenomenal they are.

Getting some adoration from others could seem like the simplest method for supporting your mental self view, however you should work on giving some affection first.

Hyping up great characteristics about others will assist you with appearing to be seriously engaging in their eyes and cause you to understand the beneficial things about yourself, as well. Concentrate on uncovered that men who utilized analogies to praise ladies were viewed as more appealing.

"Figuring out how to appropriately commend may simply be the way in to a subsequent date." "Helping others have a positive outlook on themselves expands your engaging quality. People put effort into planning for a date so carve out a time to compliment the other individual and wouldn't kid about this!"

Put a grin on.

Try not to misjudge a decent grin.

No mystery grinning causes you to appear to be warm and welcoming to others, which can assist how they with seeing you. Be that as it may, it turns out you might try and get similar advantages by thoroughly searching in a mirror and grinning at yourself.

"As amicable creatures, we are adjusted to see the non-verbal correspondence of others and clear for prompts of safety and welcome."

"Grinning is a general sign for warmth, receptiveness, and engaging quality."

"However, this likewise works independently; on the off chance that you grin at yourself in the mirror, you get very much like brain signs as you would assuming a recognizable companion grinned at you."

Specialists concentrated on what looks can mean for an individual's state of mind and found proof that recommends individuals who grin more can really feel more joyful.

Give yourself a motivational speech.

It might feel senseless, yet it can work.

It's consistently decent when somebody near you notification or brings up a decent quality, yet you don't need to sit around idly for that additional lift.

It might appear to be senseless, yet rehashing positive assertions to yourself in the mirror or making statements that you like about yourself will assist you with approving those qualities and worth them in yourself.

"Thought is a training in conscious focus," Francis said. "Anything you focus completely on will stretch out in your field of comprehension.

Finding opportunity to effectively see positive characteristics about yourself, whether outside attributes or inward abilities and characteristics, assists them with turning out to be more notable to you. At the point when you invest energy recognizing these qualities, you can encounter them all the more completely."

It is proposed that individuals who conversed with themselves had higher work achievement and certainty. Tests showed that when individuals conversed with themselves — similarly that they would address a companion — it advertised them up. The concentrate likewise showed that individuals infused more energy into giving the signal "you" while alluding to themselves.

Don't behave destructively.

Recognize what propensities are holding you up.

A review uncovered that individuals who harped on bad perspectives about themselves really had a higher gamble of self-question and may have a lower-pace of smugness.

On the off chance that you end up offering negative expressions about yourself, you want to give close consideration to why. These sorts of assertions can exacerbate you about yourself and negatively affect your mental self view.

Analyst suggests that individuals distinguish what is making them offer these expressions and dispose of the reason in the event that they would be able.

"Specifically, really focus on what triggers behaving destructively explanations." "Is it a specific climate? Individual? Circumstance? When you recognize the triggers of negative self-talk, you have a superior possibility getting yourself, transforming negative self-explanations into positive ones, and in any event, forestalling them."

Try not to offer critical remarks.

In the event that you judge others, it's likely adversely affecting your fearlessness.

Like negative self-talk, talking and considering ineffectively others can diminish your general certainty, specialists say.

At the point when we judge others, it frequently comes from a position of looking for security when we can't have a deep understanding of another person, However being excessively critical can build sensations of uneasiness and sadness and really exacerbate us about ourselves generally speaking, as per a February 2019 concentrate in the diary Character and Individual Contrasts.

That is the reason Dorrance Corridor proposed getting in the act of assuming the best about individuals when you want to bounce into judgment mode.

Evaluate your associations with others.

Eliminate the hurtful people in your everyday presence.

The heaviness of a poisonous individual in your life might be keeping you from feeling your best.

Concentrates on studied individuals who had a relationship in their life that displayed characteristics of "alienation, change, mixed up fellowship, and misleading kinship." The investigation discovered that they frequently didn't understand that others were hauling them down and owned harmful individuals "rose-hued glasses," which can negatively affect their emotional well-being.

Assuming there are individuals who are continually putting you down, being discourteous to you, or are simply terrible impacts on your confidence, put forth a valiant effort to remove those individuals of your life or invest less energy with them.

All the more significantly, focus on individuals who invest their energy supporting you and developing you. This can immediately help your certainty, De Luca said.

Have a funny bone.

Go ahead and dismiss it.

Giggling and kidding can make you more calm, so assuming that you attempt and ignore something seemingly insignificant that would regularly get under your skin, you can ease the heat off of yourself, which can make you see yourself in a positive light.

"This is so huge — certain people treat each piece of their life so truly and this shows directly before them and in their personality."

"It is entirely OK to be defective — nobody must be ideal constantly. It is significant not to allow others to characterize you and to simply be you."

Telling a wisecrack can help other people see you as more alluring, as well.

A recent report by the College of Kansas found that giggling together can increment fascination in couples. In the review, 51 sets of individuals who didn't have the foggiest idea about one another talked; the more times a man attempted to be entertaining and the more times a woman giggled at his jokes, the more plausible she was earnestly enthused about him.

Also, the more the pair snickered together, the more elevated level of fascination they revealed.

Engage in sexual relations.

Not that you really wanted a reason!

Having intercourse is an extraordinary, fun, and quite simple method for supporting your mental self portrait.

Individuals who had easygoing sex with a strong accomplice were found to show an expansion in certainty and mental self portrait, as per a recent report from the "Diary of Social Mental and Character Science."

Additionally, the pheromones you discharge during and after sex can naturally attract individuals to you, making you more alluring to them as well, as per research led by San Francisco State College.

Counterfeit it until you make it.

Carry on like you are the most certain individual in the room.

The simplest method for causing yourself to feel sure? Carry on like you as of now are.

At the point when you challenge yourself to feel far better about yourself, it will show and others will pay heed.

"How you go into a room or deal a look are characteristics of your conviction working for you or against you." "Everything unquestionably revolves around your grin, non-verbal communication and even eye to eye connection. At the point when you feel odd or off-kilter individuals can get on that disquiet which will liken to whether you are seen as alluring."

Need some motivation? A recent report distributed in the "Diary of Exploratory Social Brain science" found that basically reviewing a second when you were sure can expand levels of self-assurance.

Rock some red.

This tone can consequently cause you to feel more blazing.

Having a closet that causes you to feel sure is a gigantic move toward driving up how you see yourself, yet resting easier thinking about your appearance might be basically as straightforward as wearing an alternate tone.

A review recommends that wearing red can consequently make ladies more alluring to men. They were more likely in the survey to ask out a woman wearing a red shirt than one in green.

Red "addresses energy, power and hotness." She endorses shaking red to be dealt with more in a serious manner and to get a flood of reinforcing for yourself.

Stand upright and tall.

Further developing your stance can change your contemplations.

Having great stance can do right by you, however it can likewise encourage you.

Investigation discovered that sitting upright can cause you to feel more sure and strong. They found that individuals who strike "power presents" detailed heights in testosterone, diminishes in cortisol (a synthetic found when you experience dread), and expanded sensations of force.

Thus, in the event that you're searching for a mind-set support and to see yourself in a more sure light, it very well may merit staying cheerful both genuinely and intellectually.

CONCLUSION

The most appealing individuals on the planet have just what you have. They are people being, whatever and whoever they came here to be. All things considered, to encounter more love, euphoria and bliss in your life, then, at that point, draw in that. If you have any desire to be in a blissful, cherishing relationship, draw in that. Ideally, with these 7 hints, you can show up more appealing than you truly are. Since, the more alluring you are, the better possibilities you'll have at drawing in who you need, and what you need.

• In dating, it is about actual accessibility: "Will this individual mate with me?"

• With companions and long haul significant others, it is about close to home accessibility: "Will this individual open dependent upon me?"

• For business, it is about monetary and scholarly accessibility: "Will this individual work with me?"

The most effective way to show accessibility — whether it is at a systems administration occasion, party, conference, or date — is by exhibiting accessibility.

Showing up isn't sufficient! You need to show individuals you are sincerely accessible to associate.

Show individuals you need to interface, talk, and begin a relationship. A lady at an occasion once asked me: "Isn't clearly I'm free to interface? I'm here, right?"

Indeed, there's a brain science term called signal enhancement inclination. More or less, signal enhancement inclination is when individuals will generally think their being a tease prompts are obvious

This implies you truly need to make your non verbals self-evident, or it's logical others won't get on them.

Activity Step: At your next get-together, try explaining to individuals why you are there and what you are searching for. Something like:

- "I'm eager to meet you since I was wanting to make a few truly fascinating associations at this occasion."

- "This occasion is going perfectly. I came needing to work up some business, and I have proactively passed out a couple of business cards. May I give you one?"

We don't understand that our accessibility isn't generally so clear as we suspect. Have a go at showing it, and you will be wonderfully shocked at how inviting and inquisitive individuals are consequently.